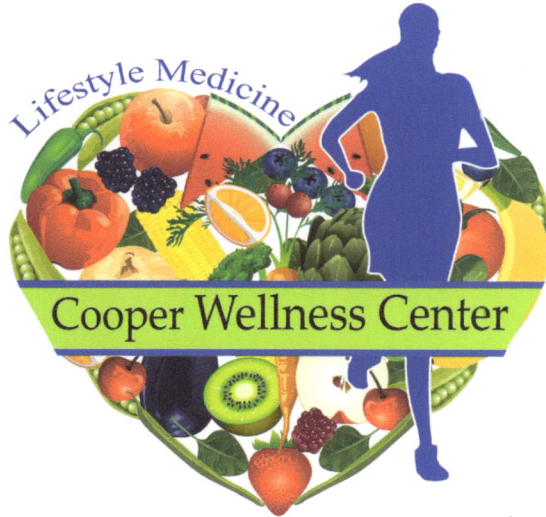

Lifestyle Medicine

Cooper Wellness Center

EXERCISE & NUTRITION
WORK MANUAL

MEDICAL DISCLAIMER:
This manual is intended to educate, inspire, and empower you to make lifestyle changes that will propel you to a healthier, happier, and more fulfilled life. You should use the information received in this manual wisely. Always consult with your primary healthcare provider if you have questions or concerns. The information presented herein should be used to supplement, not replace, medical advice from your primary healthcare provider.

The information, ideas, and suggestions in this book are not intended as a substitute for professional medical advice. Before following any suggestions contained in this book, you should consult your personal physician. Neither the author nor the publisher shall be liable or responsible for any loss or damage allegedly arising because of your use or application of any information or suggestions in this book.

Cooper Wellness and Disease Prevention Center
3604 N. McColl Rd. McAllen, TX 78501
www.CooperWellnessCenter.com

Printed in the United States of America.
ISBN: 9781733165495

CONTENTS

WELCOME TO WELLNESS!

Once again, we are excited that you have joined the Cooper Wellness and Disease Prevention Program. We are committed to preventing and reducing chronic diseases through lifestyle medicine, countless number of people have used this program and they are doing well. This book is a supplement to the Wellness Program Lecture Manual and for maximum health benefits, these books should be used together. You are to use the recipes and exercise routines as guides as you develop healthier habits.

Always remember that "good health is a choice and not a destiny", therefore in order to maintain the change for the rest of your life, do the following daily:

- ❖ Consume an abundant amount of vegetables of all colors.
- ❖ Consume four to five servings of fruits.
- ❖ Consume at least three servings of whole grains.
- ❖ Consume two to three serving of legumes.
- ❖ Add small amounts for seeds (chia, flax, pumpkin, sunflower, etc) to your meal.
- ❖ Consume a handful of nuts.
- ❖ Perform 30 minutes of moderate exercise at least 4 times per week.
- ❖ Trust God and cultivate a positive mindset.
- ❖ Drink 8 glasses of water at least.
- ❖ Sleep on average 7 to 8 hours and rest one day a week.
- ❖ Persevere until you achieve your goal.

Healthy Vegan Recipes

Most practicing physicians will confess that nutrition was not emphasized during their medical training. However, using food as medicine and focusing on a healthy lifestyle is now fast becoming the gold standard in managing patients with chronic diseases, such as diabetes, heart disease, hypertension, and even cancer.

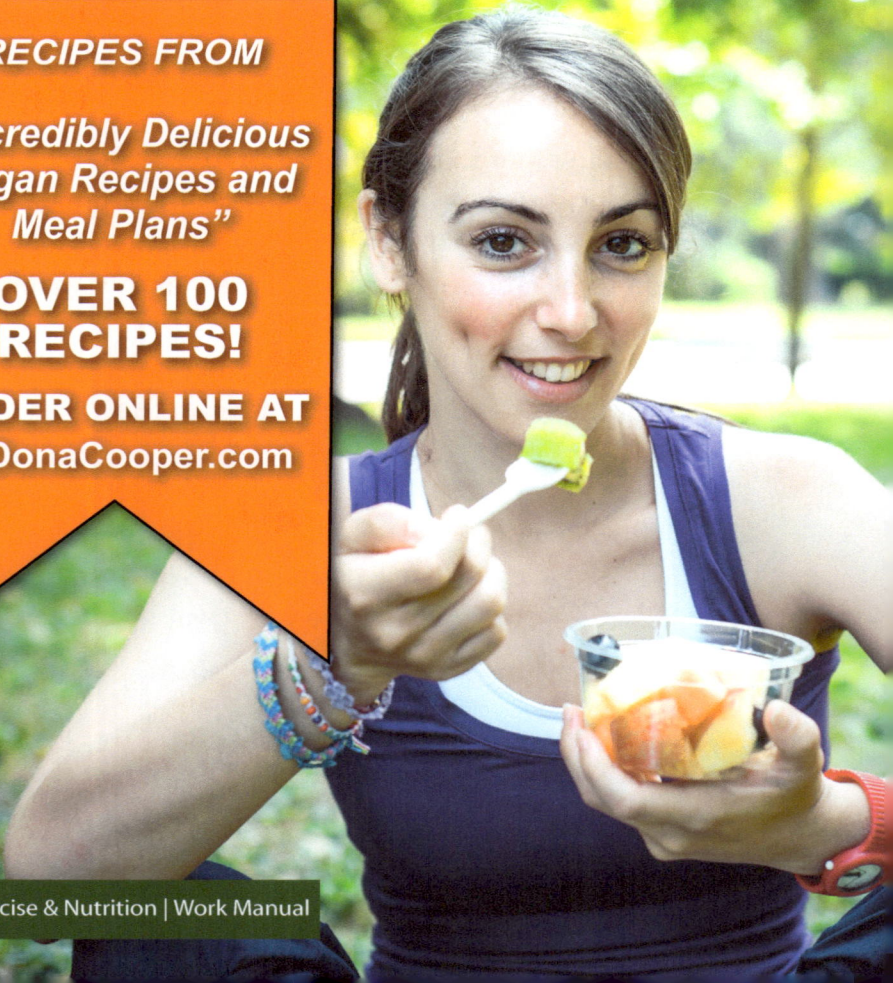

Healthy Vegan Recipes
by Dr. Dona Cooper-Dockery

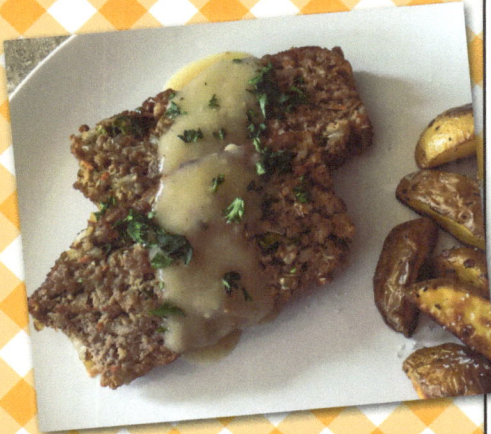

Cashew Brown Rice Loaf

2 cup cashews, raw
2 cups steamed brown rice
2 cups rich nut or soy milk
2 large onions, chopped
1 cup celery, finely chopped
¾ cup whole wheat bread crumbs
2 tablespoon Bragg's Amino Acids or soy
2 tablespoons thyme
2 teaspoons sage
2 tablespoons parsley, dried
1 teaspoon celery seed
1 teaspoon salt or to taste
1 teaspoon garlic powder
2 tablespoon nutritional yeast
2 tablespoons browning
2 tablespoons olive oil

This is quick and easy to prepare. Serve with cashew or mushroom gravy on a bed of green vegetable salad.

Place nuts and liquid ingredients in food processor or blender and chop. Add all other ingredients and continue to process. Spoon into baking loaf dish, cover with foil and bake for at least for 1 hour at 350 degrees Fahrenheit.

Eggplant Zucchini Bake

Delicious and packed with vitamins and fiber, this is dish is great for everyone but is especially ideal for diabetic or those who are trying to lose weight.

2 tablespoons olive oil
4 large zucchini (1-inch cubes)
2 medium eggplants (1-inch cubes)
2 cups cherry tomato (cut in halves)
1 small onion, chopped
1 tablespoon garlic powder
¼ cup basil, fresh
¼ cup parsley
Salt to taste

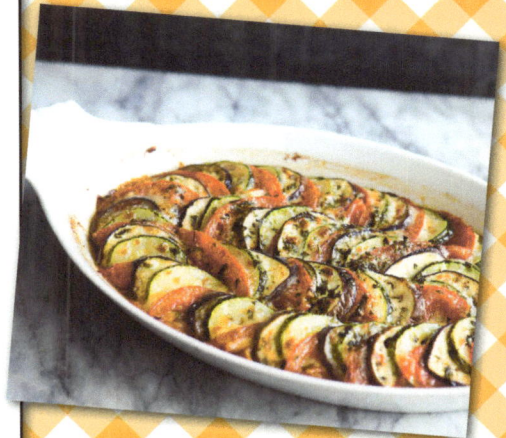

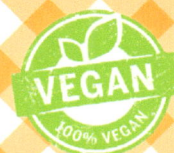

Place oil in casserole dish and add zucchini, eggplant, and cherry tomatoes. Add other ingredients. Salt to taste and mix. Bake for 30 minutes, uncovered. Then cover with foil and bake for another 15 minutes.

VEGAN
100% VEGAN

Healthy Vegan Recipes
by Dr. Dona Cooper-Dockery

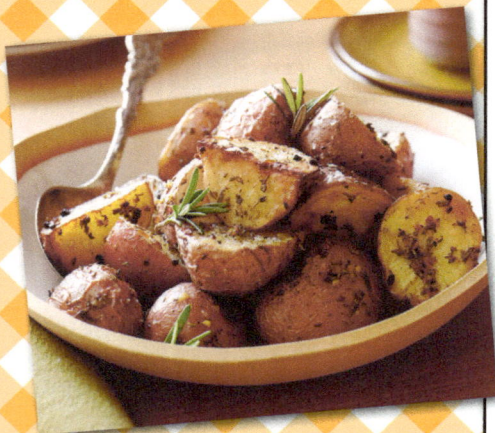

Oven Roasted Potatoes

4 lbs small red potatoes, halved
1½ tbsp olive oil
4 tsp fresh rosemary, chopped
2 tsp Mrs. Dash Seasoning
1 medium onion, chopped
2 tbsp McKay's Chicken Seasoning (Vegan)
1 tsp salt, to taste

This is a great side dish you can enjoy any time of the day. You could also add firm tofu (cubed) and bake. Makes a great main dish.

Preheat oven to 400 °F. Place potatoes in a single layer baking sheet and sprinkle oil over potatoes. Then evenly mix in all the other ingredients. Cover with foil and bake for 12-15 minutes. Remove foil and continue to bake for an additional 15 minutes or until golden brown.

Baked Falafel

Preheat the oven to 350 degrees Fahrenheit. In a food processor, add the garbanzo beans, fresh lemon juice, onion, and garlic, and puree until smooth. Put the bean mixture in a large bowl and add all the other dry seasoning (oregano, basil, cumin, cayenne, paprika, and salt). Then, stir in the bread crumbs to hold the mixture together. Add more bread crumbs if the mixture is not holding together. Roll into 1-inch balls, and place them on a cooking sheet. Lightly spray the falafel with oil and bake in the oven for 10 to 15 minutes per side or until falafel are lightly browned. Test for doneness by pressing the outside with your finger. The falafel should come out moist inside and give to the pressure of your finger.

Falafel is a well-known vegetarian dish that is served in a pita bread pocket with hummus and fresh vegetables. Feel free to add your special spices and herbs.

1 ½ (15-ounce) can garbanzo beans (chickpeas), drained, and ¼ cup liquid reserved
¼ cup fresh lemon juice
1 small onion, finely chopped
2 cloves garlic
¼ cup fresh cilantro
½ teaspoon dried basil
½ teaspoon dried oregano
1 teaspoon cumin
¼ teaspoon cayenne
½ teaspoon paprika
1 teaspoon salt
1 ½ cups whole wheat bread crumbs

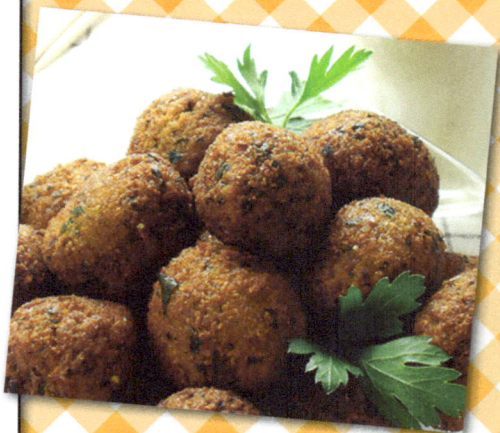

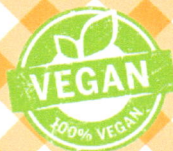

VEGAN
100% VEGAN

Healthy Vegan Recipes
by Dr. Dona Cooper-Dockery

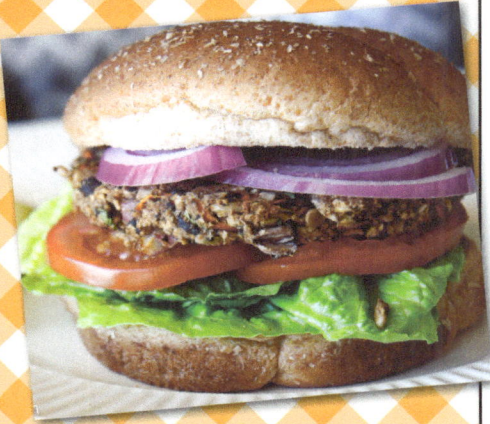

Oat-Nut Burgers

2 cups rolled oats
½ teaspoon onion powder
1 cup finely chopped walnuts
½ teaspoon coriander
½ teaspoon sage
1 tablespoon soy sauce
½ teaspoon garlic powder
½ teaspoon dried sage
1 small onion, finely chopped
2 cups hot water
1 tablespoon nutritional yeast

This burger patty is filled with fiber and good fat. Serve with tomato and lettuce on whole wheat bun or bread.

Place all of the ingredients in hot water, cover, and let rest for 20 minutes. Form into six or eight patties. Cook on a nonstick griddle over medium heat until browned on each side, 20 to 30 minutes.

Bean Burrito

This is a well-known and easy to prepare Mexican dish. These can be served at any time of the day.

Warm tortillas and spread the beans over the tortillas. Fold like an envelope. Serve with lettuce, tomato, onions, olives, and avocado and top with salsa and soy sour cream.

1 whole-wheat tortilla
¼ cup spicy Mexican beans (mashed)
Desired amount of:
Chopped lettuce
Chopped tomatoes
Diced onions
Olives
Avocado
Salsa
Soy sour cream (non-dairy)

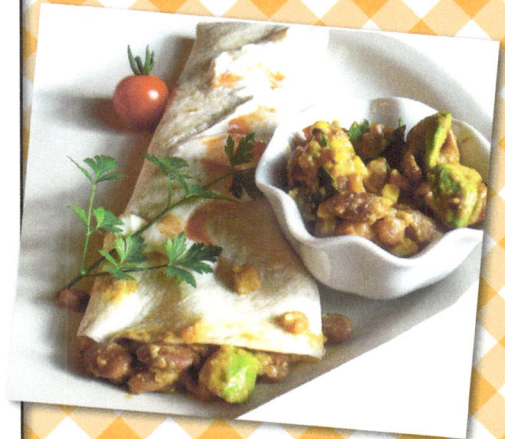

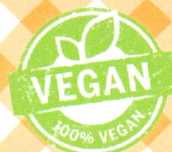

VEGAN
100% VEGAN

Healthy Vegan Recipes
by Dr. Dona Cooper-Dockery

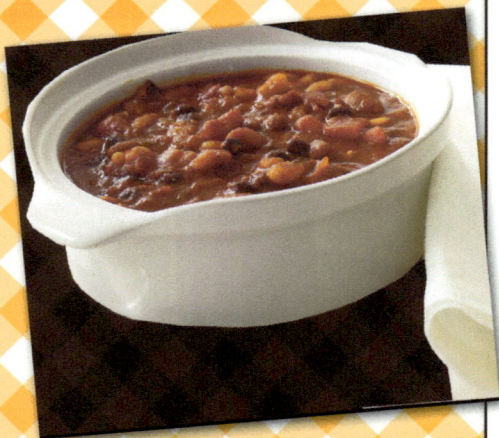

Heart-Healthy Bean Chili

1 tablespoon olive oil or vegetable oil
2 cups onions, diced
4 cloves garlic, mashed and then minced
1 cup carrot, chopped
2 cups vegetable broth
2 cups cooked kidney beans
2 cups cooked red beans
2 cups cooked black beans
1 cup frozen corn
3 cups cooked, chopped tomatoes
¾ cup of green bell pepper
1 tablespoon cumin powder
1 teaspoon dried oregano
3–4 bay leaves
1 teaspoon cayenne pepper
1 teaspoon sea salt, to taste

This dish is a great meat substitute. It is high in protein and fiber. It is ideal for those who are losing weight and will assist with keeping your blood sugar down if you are diabetic. Serve with fresh mixed vegetables or with baked sweet potato.

In a large, deep pot, add vegetable/olive oil and sauté onion, garlic, and onions for 3 to 5 minutes. Then add vegetable broth and the remaining ingredients and spices. Allow the mixture to cook for another 20 minutes.

Hummus and Veggie Wrap

This dish is very quick and easy to prepare. There are different types of tortillas that you could use: sun-dried tomato, spinach, and whole wheat. You also have the option to add your favorite veggies.

Microwave the tortilla for a few seconds to make it pliable. Spread the hummus over the tortilla, and then layer on the assorted vegetables. Wrap the tortilla like a burrito and enjoy.

2 (12-inch) whole-grain tortillas
½ cup hummus (refer to recipe on page 146)
1 cup spinach or kale
1 medium zucchini, cut in strips
1 large carrot, cut in strips
¼ cup black olives
½ cup tomato, sliced
½ cup avocado, sliced
½ cucumber, sliced

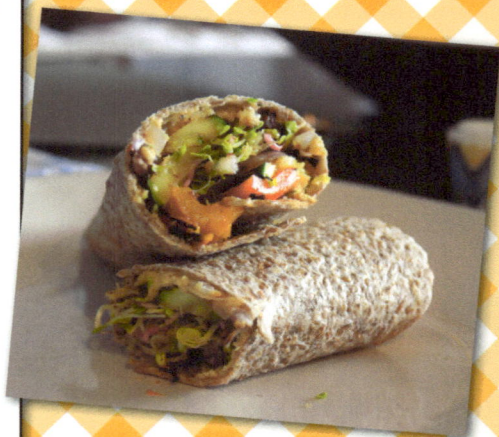

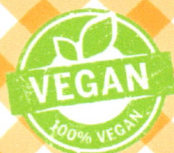

VEGAN
100% VEGAN

Healthy Vegan Recipes
by Dr. Dona Cooper-Dockery

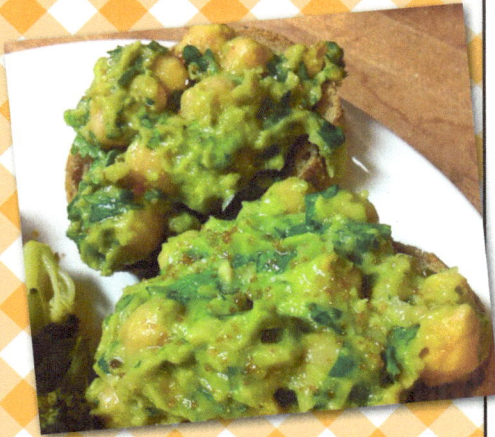

Chickpea Avocado Spread

1 medium avocado
15 ounce chickpeas
1 tablespoon lemon juice
½ sweet onion
Salt to taste

Remove peel and seed from avocado. Drain and rinse chickpeas. Add all the ingredients to the food processor and process until smooth. Can be used as sandwich spread or dip.

This spread make a wholesome and delicious sandwich. Just add tomato, spinach leaves, and alfalfa sprouts.

Seasoned Black Bean Brown Rice

If you enjoy black beans, then this is a great dish for you.

Preheat oven to 350 degrees Fahrenheit. On low heat, sauté for 2 to 3 minutes the onion and garlic in a small amount of water. Add in the rice, black beans, and other ingredients. Continue to sauté for another 3 minutes. Now add the 4 cups of water. Pour mixture in a casserole dish, cover, and place in preheated oven at 350 degrees Fahrenheit for 60 minutes. Use as a main dish or serve with a fresh vegetable salad.

1 medium onion, chopped
3 cloves garlic, mashed and diced
2 cups long-grain un-cooked brown rice
1 (15-ounce) can black beans
4 cups water
2 teaspoons thyme
1 tablespoon McKay's chicken-style seasoning
1 tablespoon Mrs. Dash, salt-free seasoning

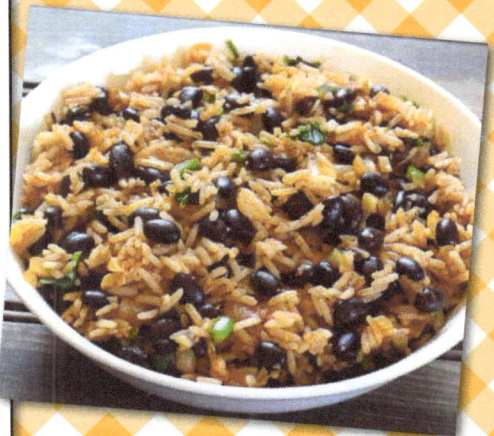

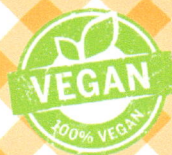

VEGAN
100% VEGAN

Healthy Vegan Recipes
by Dr. Dona Cooper-Dockery

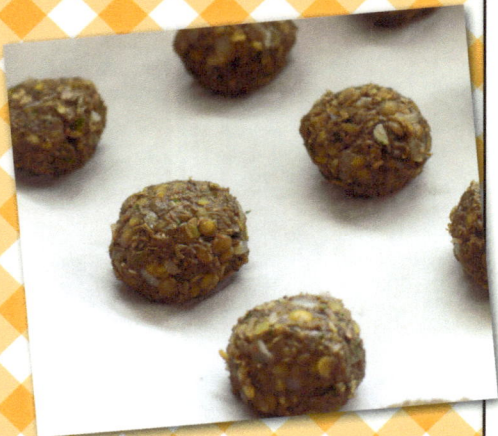

Lentil Walnut "Meatballs"

1 cup soaked lentils (cover in water and soak overnight)
¼ cup of walnuts, chopped
½ cup onion, chopped
1 teaspoon thyme
1 teaspoon cumin
2 tablespoons tahini
1 teaspoon garlic powder
½ cup oat flour
1 teaspoon sage
1 teaspoon salt
1 teaspoon fresh basil, finely chopped

These look and taste better than meat. Cook in tomato sauce and serve over whole wheat spaghetti.

Pour off the water and then blend lentil to a paste. Place lentils in a bowl. Add all the other ingredients and mix together. Form small balls and then place them on a baking tray. Preheat oven to 200 degrees Fahrenheit, and bake for approximately 20 to 25 minutes.

"Meatball" Tomato Sauce

1 ½ cup tomato puree
½ cup onion, chopped
1 clove garlic, mashed and diced
2 teaspoon sweet paprika
1 ½ teaspoon thyme, dried
1 ½ cup water
2 tablespoons fresh basil, chopped
Salt to taste

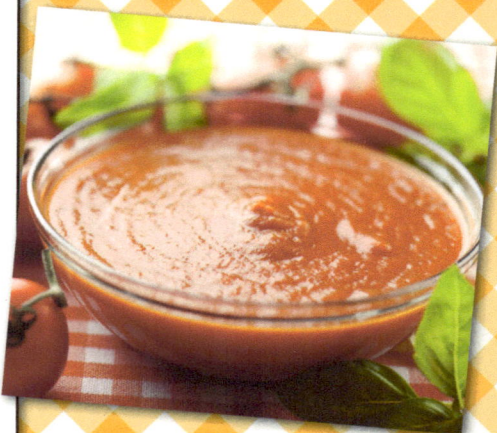

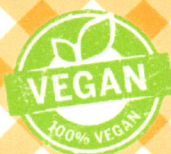

Place 2 tablespoons of water in a nonstick pan on low-to-medium heat. Add onion and garlic. Sauté for 2 to 3 minutes and add the other ingredients. Continue to sauté for another 3 minutes. Then add meatballs. Enjoy with whole-grain spaghetti.

VEGAN
100% VEGAN

Healthy Vegan Recipes
by Dr. Dona Cooper-Dockery

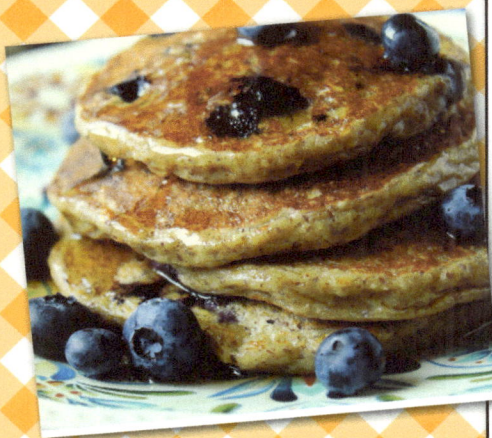

Blueberry-Oatmeal Pancakes

2 flax eggs (2 table-spoons ground flaxseed + 6 tablespoons water)
1 cup rolled oats
1 ½ cup unsweetened soy or almond milk
¼ cup walnuts
½ cup whole wheat flour
½ teaspoon baking soda
½ teaspoon baking powder
6 dates, pitted
½ teaspoon salt
1 cup fresh or frozen blueberries

These pancakes are a little denser, heartier, and more filling than the regular pancakes.

Mix ground flax with 6 tablespoons of water and let the mix stand for 10 minutes. The consistency should be that of an egg. Place oats, nuts, and milk in a blender and blend until smooth. Place mixture in bowl, and then fold in other ingredients. Add more milk if necessary for the desired consistency. Lightly grease the hot skillet or pan with additional oil. Pour ½ cup pancake rounds on the skillet and cook until bubbles form on the surface. Carefully drop 6 to 8 (optional) blueberries onto one side of each pancake, and then flip and cook on the other side until golden brown.

Toast and Gravy

If you are a lover of biscuits and gravy, then this breakfast option is for you. It is fast and easy to prepare, and, most important, it is healthy with good fats.

Place all ingredients except cornstarch in a high-speed blender with 1½ cup of water. Blend until smooth. Place mixture in a saucepan. Allow to simmer on medium heat. Mix cornstarch in remaining water and incorporate to boiling mixture. Stir frequently until smooth. Place toast bread on plate. Pour gravy over toast and enjoy!

½ cup almonds
2 cups water
2 tablespoons McKay's chicken-style seasoning
2 tablespoon Bragg's Amino Acids
1 tablespoon nutritional yeast
½ teaspoon garlic powder
½ teaspoon onion powder
1 small onion
½ teaspoon dry basil
2 tablespoons corn-starch

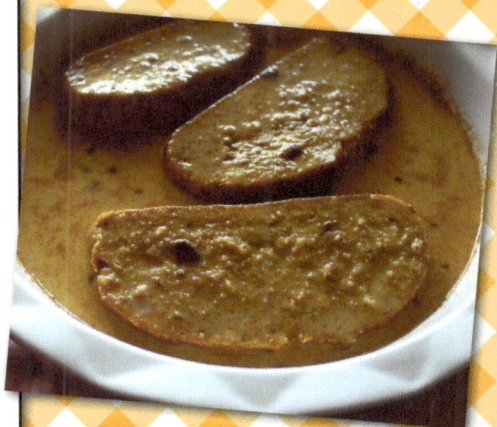

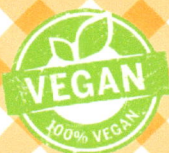

VEGAN
100% VEGAN

Healthy Vegan Recipes
by Dr. Dona Cooper-Dockery

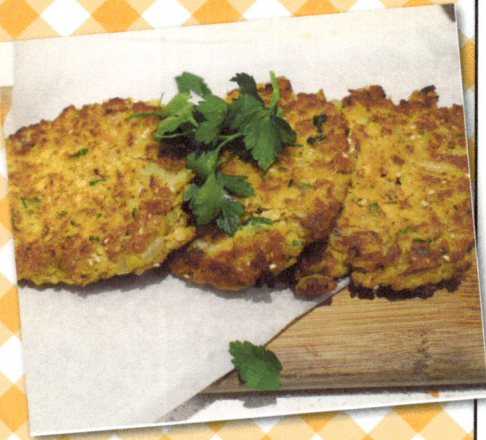

Lentil Patties

2 cups cooked red lentils, drained
½ cup onions, finely chopped
1 teaspoon dried thyme
1 cup finely ground chia seeds
¼ cup brown rice flour or oatmeal flour
2 teaspoons sea salt
1 teaspoon garlic powder
1 teaspoon onion powder
1 ¼ teaspoon sage
1 cup grated carrots
1 cup pecans
175 grams tiny mushrooms, drained and chopped
1 cup water or milk
1 cup celery, finely chopped

These are absolutely delicious. You will not miss the meat. Serve on a bun or with gravy over rice or baked potato or with mixed vegetables.

Line your baking pan with parchment paper or spray your pan with oil. Mix all the ingredients together and make patties. Put patties on the baking pan. Bake at 350 degrees Fahrenheit for 30 minutes. Turn them over after 20 minutes. Hint—use an ice cream scoop and make balls instead of patties and bake.

Jamaican Stewed Peas

This dish is high in protein and fiber and goes well with rice, potatoes, or steamed mixed veggies. A great dish for diabetics, the high fiber content promotes blood sugar control.

2 cups dry red kidney beans
1 large onion, chopped
2 stalks scallion, mashed and chopped
4 cloves garlic
3 sprigs fresh thyme, chopped
2 teaspoons savory seasoning salt
1 (15-ounce) can coconut milk
2 tablespoons vegetable or olive oil

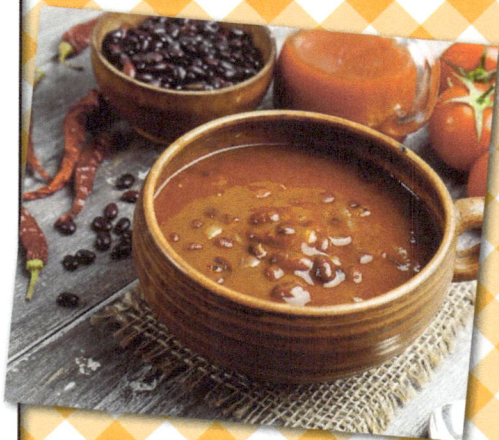

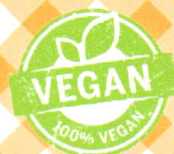

Place beans in 8 cups water and soak overnight. Pour water off. Add 6 cups water and cook for about 2 hours until tender. Add all the other ingredients and allow to simmer on low-to-medium heat for 1 hour until cooked. Serve with seasoned brown rice and fresh vegetable salad.

VEGAN
100% VEGAN

Healthy Vegan Recipes
by Dr. Dona Cooper-Dockery

Avocado Toast

4 thick slices of multi-grain bread
1 ripe avocado
¼ cup lime juice + pinch of salt
1 large sliced tomato
½ cup black beans (warmed)
½ small red onion, chopped

Mash avocado with a fork until smooth, sprinkle salt, add onion and lime juice. Toast bread, then spread the avocado and add sliced tomato and spoonful of black beans for added protein.

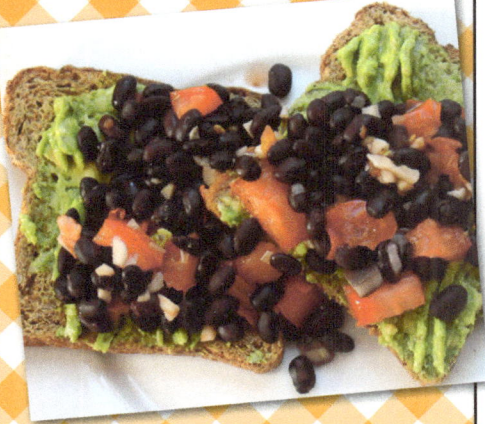

Black Bean Burger

In a medium-sized bowl, mash beans with fork and set aside. Place the onion, jalapeño, and garlic in a food processor and pulse 5to 6 times. Add oats, corn, cilantro, cumin, curry powder, and cayenne. Season to taste with salt, and pulse about 10 to 12 times. Remove ingredients from food processor and add to bowl with mashed beans and stir well. Spray a small amount of oil into a skillet and heat to medium. Form the burger mixture into 4 equal patties. Cook the patties for 5 to 7 minutes on each side or until a golden crust develops and the patties are heated through. Remove the patties from the heat and place onto burger buns. Add sliced tomato, lettuce, mustard, and ketchup.

1 (15-ounce) can black beans, drained
½ jalapeño, seeded and chopped
3 garlic cloves
½ medium onion, cut in wedges
⅔ cup rolled oats
½ cup frozen corn
1 tablespoon fresh cilantro, minced
2 teaspoon ground cumin
½ teaspoon curry powder
¼ teaspoon cayenne pepper
¼ cup bread crumbs
½ teaspoon salt or more to taste
Tomato, Mustard & Ketchup

This is a great burger to replace meat, which is high in saturated fat. If you want to keep your cholesterol down, then this is a great alternative for a healthy lunch meal.

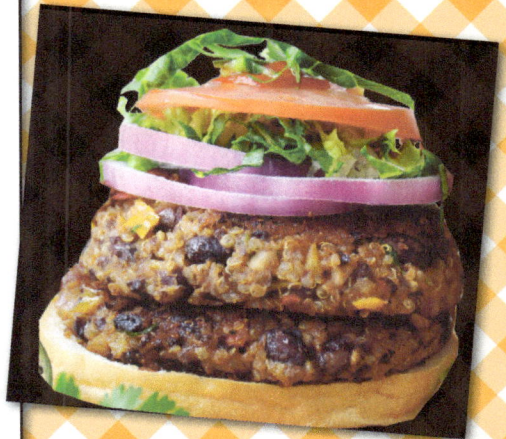

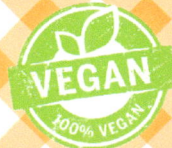

VEGAN
100% VEGAN

Healthy Vegan Recipes
by Dr. Dona Cooper-Dockery

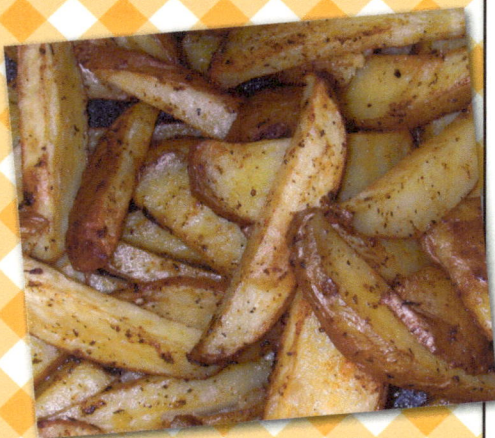

Seasoned Oven Fries

4 large potatoes
1 teaspoon Mrs. Dash
1 tablespoon McKay's seasoning
2 tablespoons soy sauce

Healthy replacement for French fries—tasty and delicious without the oil!

Slice the potatoes lengthwise. Place the potatoes in a flat baking dish. Mix all the other ingredients together then pour over the potatoes and marinate for 1 hour, turning occasionally to make sure that all are coated. Preheat oven to 450 degrees Fahrenheit. Place the potatoes on a nonstick baking sheet. Bake for 45 minutes or until lightly browned, basting occasionally with dressing.

Scrambled Tofu

Remove the tofu from its package, rinse, drain, and set aside. In large skillet/sauce pan, sauté the onion, peppers, and other spices for 5 minutes in hot oil. Scramble tofu in skillet and add remaining ingredients. Cover and allow to cook for another 10 minutes. Serve as filling for taco or with whole-wheat bread.

1 (16-oz) package water-packed, extra-firm organic tofu
½ cup chopped onion
¼ cup bell peppers
½ cup tomatoes
2 tsp McKay's Chicken Seasoning (Vegan)
½ tsp turmeric powder
½ tsp salt
½ tsp onion powder
½ tsp garlic powder
½ tsp thyme
1 tsp Mrs. Dash Seasoning
2 tsp vegetable oil

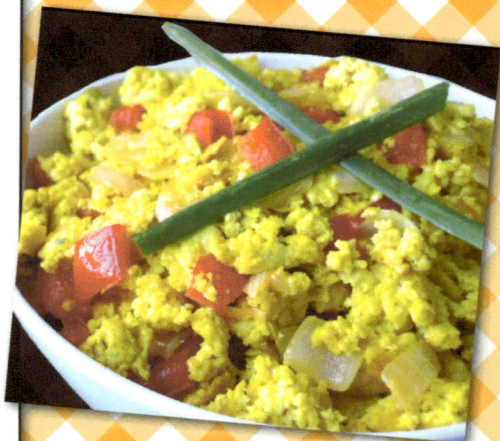

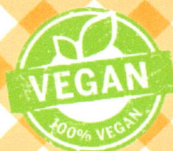

VEGAN
100% VEGAN

Healthy Vegan Recipes
by Dr. Dona Cooper-Dockery

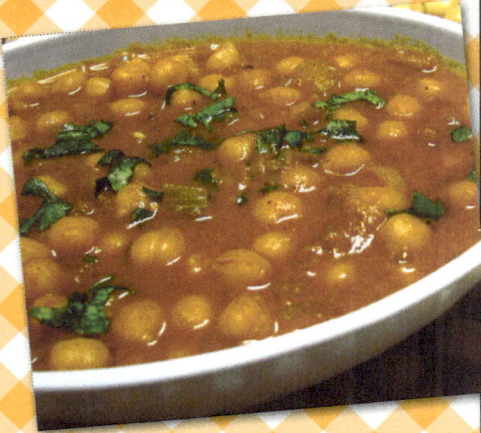

Chickpea Curry

½ cup water
1 onion minced
2 cloves garlic, minced
1 tbsp fresh ginger root, finely chopped
2 tsp cumin
1tsp ground coriander
Sea salt to taste
1 tsp cayenne pepper
1 tsp ground turmeric
2 (15 ounce) cans garbanzo beans
1 cup chopped fresh cilantro
2 tbsp olive oil

Heat oil in a large frying pan over medium heat. Add onions and spices. Sauté until tender. Then add beans and water. Cook for 20 min.

Banana Whole-Wheat Muffins

Preheat oven to 400°F. Line 12 muffin tin with paper baking cups or grease bottoms. Stir together whole-wheat flour, baking soda, salt, and nutmeg in a medium bowl. Mix crushed pineapple, milk, and banana in a large bowl. Stir in a flour mixture just until moistened (batter will be lumpy). Fold in pecans. Divide batter evenly among muffin cups. Bake 18-20 minutes or until golden brown and toothpick inserted into center comes out clean. Remove from pan to wire rack. Serve warm.

1¾ cups whole-wheat flour
2 tsp baking soda
¼ tsp salt
¼ tsp ground nutmeg
⅔ cup crushed pineapple
⅔ cup almond milk
½ cup mashed very ripe banana
1 tsp vanilla
½ cup raisins
¼ cup chopped pecans

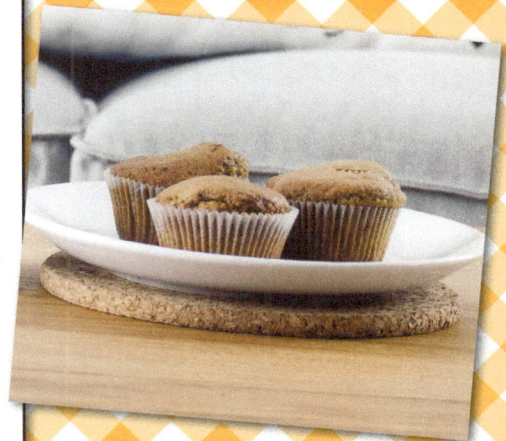

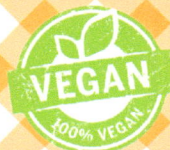

VEGAN
100% VEGAN

Healthy Vegan Recipes
by Dr. Dona Cooper-Dockery

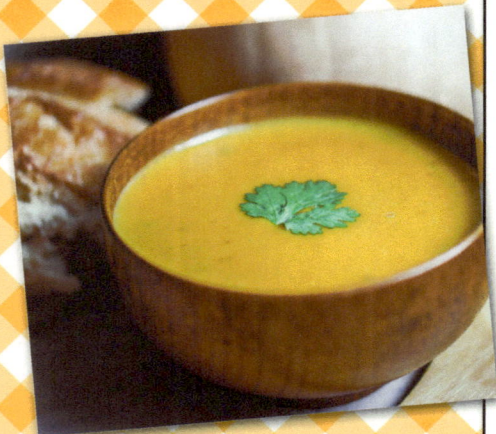

Cream of Pumpkin Soup

2 cups (1 lb) boiled
puréed pumpkin
2 cups soy milk
3 tbsp whole grain flour
1 tbsp olive oil
1 medium onion,
chopped
1 tsp Mrs. Dash
Seasoning
Salt to taste

On low heat, sauté onion in hot oil for 2 minutes. Add flour and Mrs. Dash. Then add milk slowly and continue to stir until smooth and thickened. Combine pumpkin with mixture, simmer for 5 minutes. Serve hot.

Mashed Cauliflower and White Beans

In a medium-sized pot, cook cauliflower for about 6 minutes. Pat dry with a paper towel and do not allow the cauliflower to become cold. Warm the beans on medium heat, then place in food processor with the cashews. Process for a few minutes. Add cauliflower and continue to process until smooth.

8 cups cauliflower
florets, fresh or frozen
1 (15-oz) can white or
lima beans
⅔ cup of cashews, raw
(optional)
2 tsp onion powder
2 tsp garlic powder

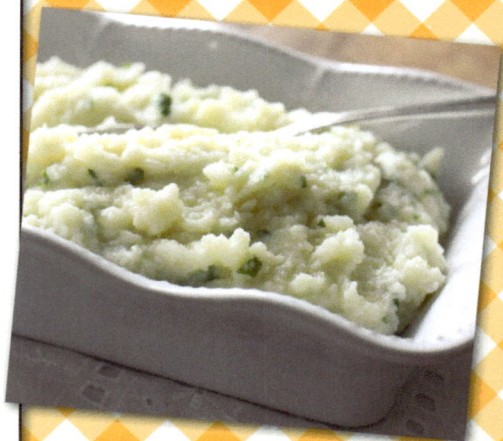

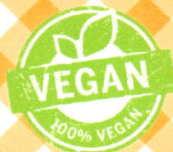

VEGAN
100% VEGAN

Healthy Vegan Recipes
by Dr. Dona Cooper-Dockery

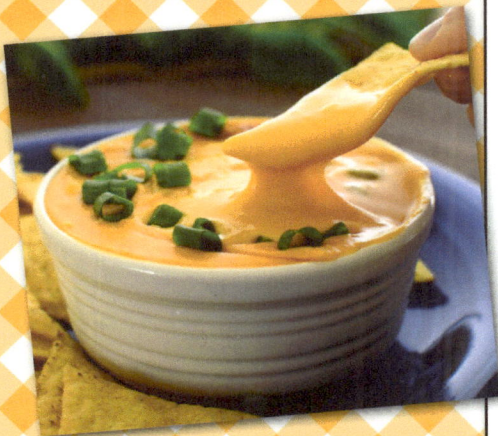

Vegan "Cheese" Sauce

½ cup raw cashew nuts (raw)
3 tbsp nutritional yeast flakes
2 cups water
2 tbsp corn starch
1 tbsp fresh lemon juice
¼ tsp garlic powder
1 large medium red bell pepper
1 ½ tsp salt
½ tsp onion powder

Blend cashew nuts in ½ cup water until smooth, add the remaining ingredients and blend until smooth. Add sauce to sauce pan and cook for 5-7 minutes on low heat, stir continuously until thickened. Remove from heat and enjoy. May use as a dip, spread or for macaroni and cheese.

Chile and Lime Quinoa

Place quinoa in fine-mesh strainer rinse well under cold running water. Combine quinoa and 1 cup water in small saucepan; Bring to a boil over high heat. Reduce heat to low, cover and simmer 12-15 minutes or until quinoa is tender. Drain, Cover, let stand 5 minutes. Stir jalapeno, green onion, oil, lime juice, salt, cumin, chili powder and Mrs Dash into quinoa. Fluff mixture with fork. Serve warm or at room temperature.

½ cup quinoa
1 small jalapeno pepper minced
2 tbsp finely chopped green onion
2 tbsp olive oil
1 tbsp fresh lime juice
¼ tsp salt
¼ tsp cumin
¼ tsp chili powder
1/8 tsp Mrs Dash

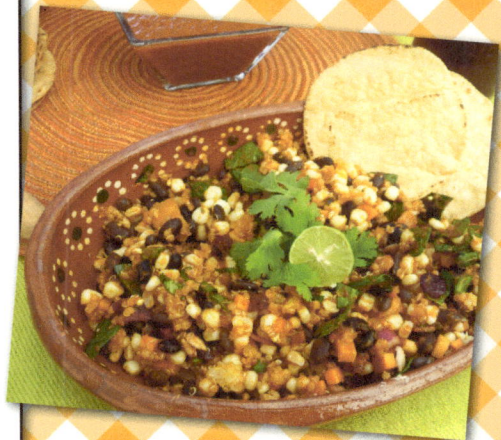

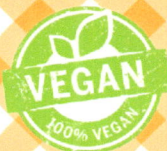

VEGAN
100% VEGAN

Healthy Vegan Recipes
by Dr. Dona Cooper-Dockery

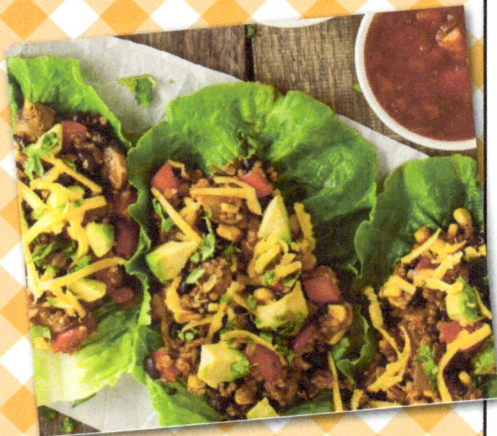

Lettuce Wraps

Red bell pepper
½ cup carrots diced
Tofu (Firm)
Soy crumbles
½ cup celery diced
4 cloves garlic
2 tbsp minced ginger
4 green onions
1 small can water chestnuts
Lettuce leaves

Sauce:
1 tbsp rice vinegar
1 tbsp sesame oil
1/3 cup teriyaki sauce

Add sesame oil to a skillet, add garlic and ginger cook and stir 2 minutes, add carrots, celery, bell pepper. Add Tofu and crumbles cook another 6 to 8 minutes, add sauce, chopped water chestnuts, and green onions. Serve on lettuce leaves and top with peanuts or cashew pieces.

Breakfast Quinoa Bowl

2 cups vanilla flavored soy or almond milk
1 cup quinoa, rinsed
1/3 cup raisins
Pinch of ground cinnamon
1 cup fresh or frozen fruit
2 tbsp of walnuts

In a small saucepan, bring milk to boil. Add quinoa and reduce the heat to simmer and cover until milk is almost absorbed, approximately 15 minutes. Stir in the cinnamon, fruit, and cook another 2-3 minutes. Sprinkle with toasted nuts.

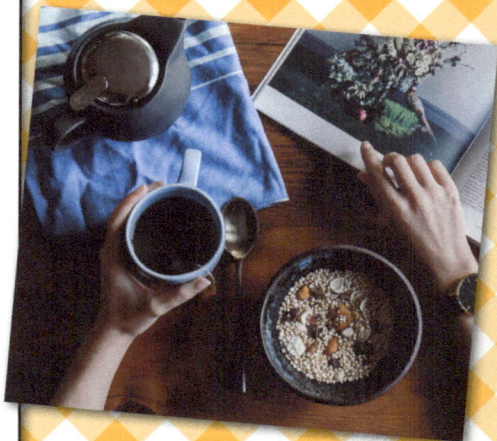

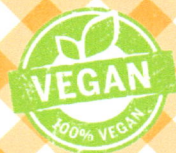

VEGAN
100% VEGAN

Healthy Vegan Recipes
by Dr. Dona Cooper-Dockery

Mushroom and Kale Frittata

1 small onion, chopped
2 cups mushrooms
2 cups Tofu Scramble
4 cups coarsely chopped kale leaves
2 cloves garlic, mashed & minced
¼ tsp salt
1 cup rolled oats
1 cup soy milk
½ cup whole-wheat flour
½ tsp baking powder
2 tbsp olive oil

Blend oats; add in wheat flour, baking powder, baking soda and salt. In a separate bowl mix milk and oil. Then combine both and set aside. Spray large oven proof skillet with nonstick cooking spray; heat over medium heat. Add onion and mushrooms; cook and stir 6-8 minutes or until onion is light golden. Add kale and garlic; cook 3-5 minutes or until kale is wilted. Evenly spread mixture to cover bottom of skillet. Pour Tofu Scramble over Kale mixture. Cover and cook 6-7 minutes or until almost set. Then mix milk, oats, flour and baking powder. Pour mixture over sautéed vegetable tofu, slightly mix. Preheat broiler. Uncover skillet; broil 2-3 minutes or until golden brown and set. Let stand 5 minutes before cutting into 6 wedges.

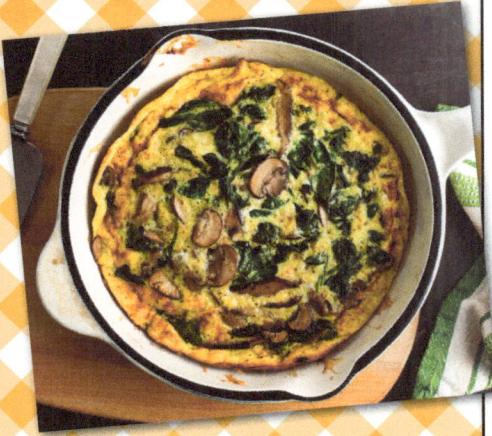

Roasted Vegetable Delight

1 green zucchini
1 yellow zucchini
3 cups broccoli
3 cups cauliflower
1 cup carrots
1 cup red pepper
½ cup diced onion
8 oz firm tofu
2 tbsp Bragg Liquid Aminos or soy sauce
1 package Lipton onion soup mix

All vegetables and tofu should be cut into small bite size pieces. Mix together all the ingredients in a large baking dish, cover and bake at 400°F for 10 minutes. Open and mix ingredients together then bake for another 10-15 minutes.

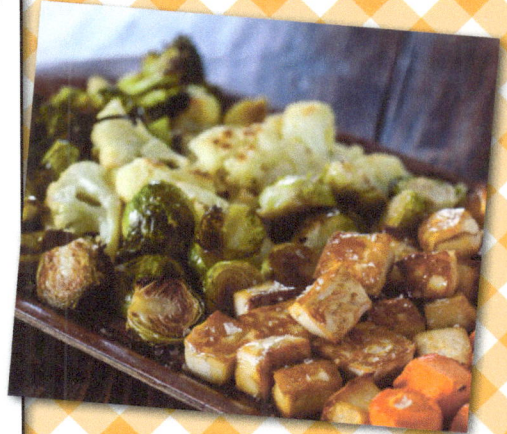

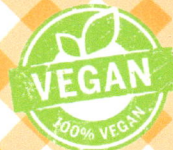

VEGAN
100% VEGAN

Healthy Vegan Recipes
by Dr. Dona Cooper-Dockery

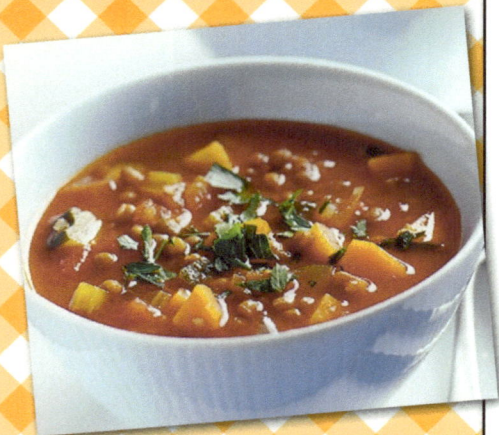

Lentil Soup with Vegetables

2 cups lentils
1½ cups onion, chopped
2 cups carrots, cubed
2 large potatoes, cubed
8 cups water
½ cup celery, chopped
2 tbsp savory seasoning
4 garlic cloves, minced
1 bay leaf
2 tsp Italian herbs or Mrs. Dash Seasoning
1 tsp thyme

In a large pot combine the lentils and water and allow to cook for about 60 minutes or until lentils are tender. Add the vegetables and all the other ingredients. Allow to cook for another 30 minutes, stirring occasionally. Serve hot.

Oatmeal Fruit Smoothie

2 cups of water, soy milk or almond milk
1 cup oatmeal (rolled oats)
1/2 frozen banana
4 frozen strawberries

Add spinach & kale leaves if you would like to make green smoothie version.

Blend all ingredients until smooth.

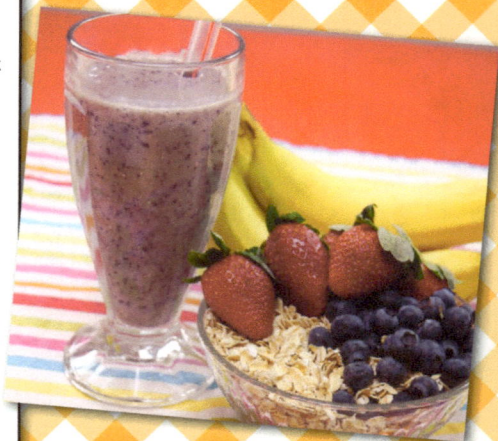

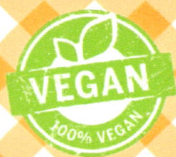

Healthy Vegan Recipes
by Dr. Dona Cooper-Dockery

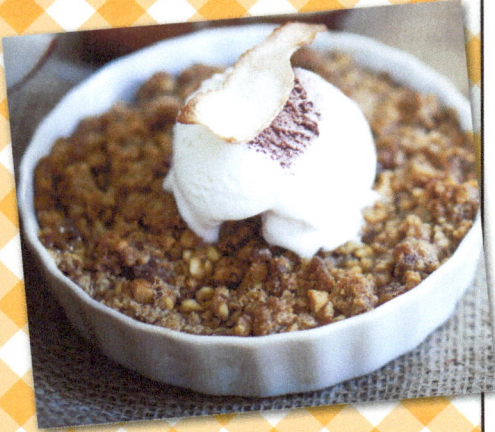

Baked Oats

2 cups rolled oats
¼ cup raisins
¼ cup dates, chopped
1 tsp ground cinnamon
1 tsp baking powder
1 cup soy/almond milk
½ cup blended apple
1 tsp vanilla extract
½ cup almond slivers

Preheat oven to 350°F. Mix all dry ingredients in a bowl, add the wet ingredients and mix well. Place mixture in a lightly oiled baking dish, spread evenly, cover and bake for 25-30 minutes. Serve warm or cold.

Coconut Curry Eggplant

Sauté curry powder and turmeric in coconut milk on low heat for 1-2 minutes. Add onion, garlic and bell pepper and simmer for another 2 minutes. Add eggplant and the remaining ingredients. Allow to cook on low-medium heat for 30 minutes or until cooked. Serve with cooked brown rice or may blend and use as a sauce which may be poured over cooked pasta.

2 large eggplants, cut in large cubes
½ cup coconut milk
2 tsp turmeric powder
2 tsp curry powder
1 medium onion, chopped
3 cloves of garlic, mashed and diced
1 tsp thyme
1 medium green bell pepper, diced
2 tsp savory seasoning salt
1 tsp salt, to taste

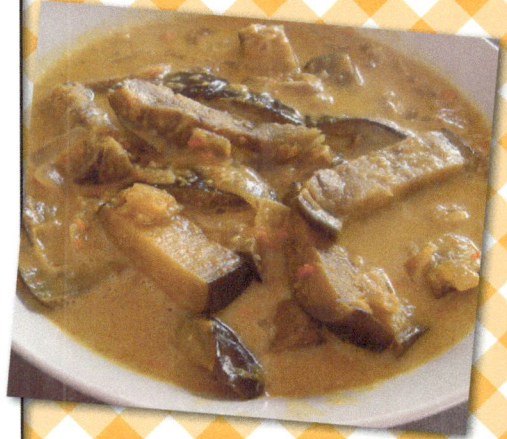

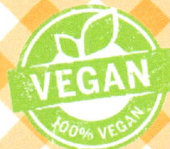

VEGAN
100% VEGAN

Healthy Vegan Recipes
by Dr. Dona Cooper-Dockery

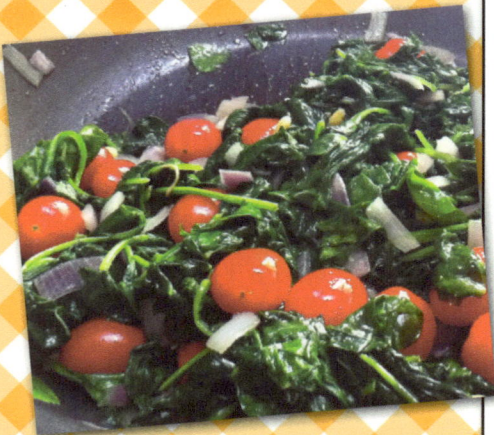

Steamed Spinach

2 (10-oz) packages frozen spinach
½ medium onion, chopped
1 small tomato, chopped
½ medium green bell pepper, chopped
2 sprigs fresh thyme
1 tsp McKay's Chicken Seasoning (Vegan)
1 tbsp olive oil

Place oil in saucepan on low-medium heat. Sauté onion, bell pepper and tomato for 3-5 minutes. Remove water from spinach and then add to saucepan. Add remaining ingredients, allow to simmer for another 7-10 minutes, taste and add extra seasoning or salt if desired. Serve with oven roasted potatoes.

Black Bean, Corn and Quinoa Salad

Over medium heat, heat oil in a saucepan and sauté the onion and garlic until they're soft and translucent. Add the quinoa to the pan and cover with vegetable broth. Season with cumin, cayenne pepper, and salt, then bring the mixture to a boil. Cover, reduce the heat and simmer for 20 minutes, stirring occasionally. Add the frozen corn to the pan and continue to simmer for 5 more minutes. Mix in the black beans, cilantro, lime juice, and optional jalapeno and cook until beans are heated through.

¼ cup quinoa, uncooked
2 (15-oz) cans black beans, rinsed and drained
½ cup fresh cilantro chopped
1 tbsp extra-virgin olive oil
1 onion, chopped
3 cloves garlic, minced
2 tbsp lime or lemon juice
1½ cups vegetable broth (low sodium)
1 jalapeno seeded and diced finely (optional)
1 tbsp ground cumin
¼ tbsp cayenne pepper
Salt to taste
2 cups frozen corn kernels

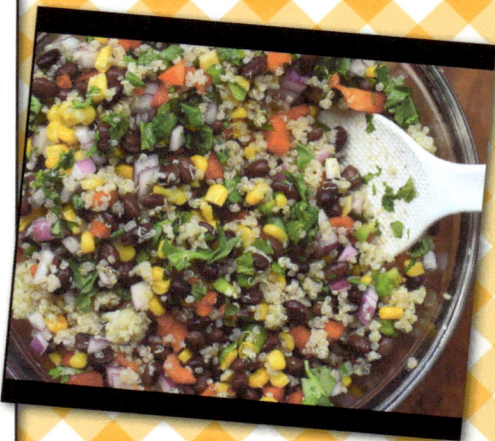

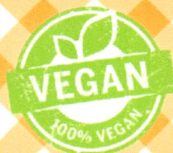

VEGAN
100% VEGAN

NOTES:

_____
_____
_____
_____
_____
_____
_____
_____
_____
_____
_____
_____
_____
_____
_____
_____
_____
_____

Meal Log — Week 1

	BREAKFAST	LUNCH	DINNER
SUN			
MON			
TUE			
WED			
THU			
FRI			
SAT			

Meal Log — Week 2

	BREAKFAST	LUNCH	DINNER
SUN			
MON			
TUE			
WED			
THU			
FRI			
SAT			

Meal Log — Week 3

	BREAKFAST	LUNCH	DINNER
SUN			
MON			
TUE			
WED			
THU			
FRI			
SAT			

Meal Log — Week 4

	BREAKFAST	LUNCH	DINNER
SUN			
MON			
TUE			
WED			
THU			
FRI			
SAT			

Meal Log — Week 5

	BREAKFAST	LUNCH	DINNER
SUN			
MON			
TUE			
WED			
THU			
FRI			
SAT			

Meal Log — Week 6

	BREAKFAST	LUNCH	DINNER
SUN			
MON			
TUE			
WED			
THU			
FRI			
SAT			

Meal Log — Week 7

	BREAKFAST	LUNCH	DINNER
SUN			
MON			
TUE			
WED			
THU			
FRI			
SAT			

Meal Log — Week 8

	BREAKFAST	LUNCH	DINNER
SUN			
MON			
TUE			
WED			
THU			
FRI			
SAT			

Personal Wellness Log — Week 1

	SUN	MON	TUE	WED	THU	FRI	SAT	T
SLEEP 7-8 hrs/day 2pts for each day achieved								
WATER 6-8 glasses/day 2pts for every day achieved								
PHYSICAL ACTIVITY 30-60 min/day 2pts for every 15 min/day								
PERSONAL GOAL _____ 2pts for each day you meet your goal								
HEALTHY FATS 1 pt/item/day, 4pts max • eat healthy fats including 1 serving of nuts daily • avoid all trans fats • limit saturated fat (less than 7% of cal.) • eat a food high in n-3 fatty acids (flax meal 1T, walnuts 1oz., canola oil 1T)								
HEALTHY CARBOHYDRATES 1 pt/item/day, 4pts max • eat 5+ servings of fruits and vegetables • eat 3+ servings of whole grains (1 slice bread, 1/2 C dry cereal) • eat a serving (1/2C) of legumes or tofu • limit high glycemic foods (pop, white bread, French fries, white rice, pastry, etc.)								
HEALTHY WEIGHT 4 pts for each day you follow a healthy, low calorie eating plan								

TOTAL WELLNESS POINTS THIS WEEK: _____

TOTAL MILES WALKED THIS WEEK: _____

Personal Wellness Log — Week 2

	SUN	MON	TUE	WED	THU	FRI	SAT	T
SLEEP 7-8 hrs/day 2pts for each day achieved								
WATER 6-8 glasses/day 2pts for every day achieved								
PHYSICAL ACTIVITY 30-60 min/day 2pts for every 15 min/day								
PERSONAL GOAL _____ 2pts for each day you meet your goal								
HEALTHY FATS 1 pt/item/day, 4pts max • eat healthy fats including 1 serving of nuts daily • avoid all trans fats • limit saturated fat (less than 7% of cal.) • eat a food high in n-3 fatty acids (flax meal 1T, walnuts 1oz., fish 2oz., canola oil 1T)								
HEALTHY CARBOHYDRATES 1 pt/item/day, 4pts max • eat 5+ servings of fruits and vegetables • eat 3+ servings of whole grains (1 slice bread, 1/2 C dry cereal) • eat a serving (1/2C) of legumes or tofu • limit high glycemic foods (pop, white bread, French fries, white rice, pastry, etc.)								
HEALTHY WEIGHT 4 pts for each day you follow a healthy, low calorie eating plan								

TOTAL WELLNESS POINTS THIS WEEK:_____

TOTAL MILES WALKED THIS WEEK: _____

Personal Wellness Log — Week 3

	SUN	MON	TUE	WED	THU	FRI	SAT	T
SLEEP 7-8 hrs/day 2pts for each day achieved								
WATER 6-8 glasses/day 2pts for every day achieved								
PHYSICAL ACTIVITY 30-60 min/day 2pts for every 15 min/day								
PERSONAL GOAL _____ 2pts for each day you meet your goal								
HEALTHY FATS 1 pt/item/day, 4pts max • eat healthy fats including 1 serving of nuts daily • avoid all trans fats • limit saturated fat (less than 7% of cal.) • eat a food high in n-3 fatty acids (flax meal 1T, walnuts 1oz., fish 2oz., canola oil 1T)								
HEALTHY CARBOHYDRATES 1 pt/item/day, 4pts max • eat 5+ servings of fruits and vegetables • eat 3+ servings of whole grains (1 slice bread, 1/2 C dry cereal) • eat a serving (1/2C) of legumes or tofu • limit high glycemic foods (pop, white bread, French fries, white rice, pastry, etc.)								
HEALTHY WEIGHT 4 pts for each day you follow a healthy, low calorie eating plan								

TOTAL WELLNESS POINTS THIS WEEK: _____

TOTAL MILES WALKED THIS WEEK: _____

Personal Wellness Log — Week 4

	SUN	MON	TUE	WED	THU	FRI	SAT	T
SLEEP 7-8 hrs/day 2pts for each day achieved								
WATER 6-8 glasses/day 2pts for every day achieved								
PHYSICAL ACTIVITY 30-60 min/day 2pts for every 15 min/day								
PERSONAL GOAL _____ 2pts for each day you meet your goal								
HEALTHY FATS 1 pt/item/day, 4pts max • eat healthy fats including 1 serving of nuts daily • avoid all trans fats • limit saturated fat (less than 7% of cal.) • eat a food high in n-3 fatty acids (flax meal 1T, walnuts 1oz., fish 2oz., canola oil 1T)								
HEALTHY CARBOHYDRATES 1 pt/item/day, 4pts max • eat 5+ servings of fruits and vegetables • eat 3+ servings of whole grains (1 slice bread, 1/2 C dry cereal) • eat a serving (1/2C) of legumes or tofu • limit high glycemic foods (pop, white bread, French fries, white rice, pastry, etc.)								
HEALTHY WEIGHT 4 pts for each day you follow a healthy, low calorie eating plan								

TOTAL WELLNESS POINTS THIS WEEK:_____

TOTAL MILES WALKED THIS WEEK: _____

Personal Wellness Log — Week 5

	SUN	MON	TUE	WED	THU	FRI	SAT	T
SLEEP 7-8 hrs/day 2pts for each day achieved								
WATER 6-8 glasses/day 2pts for every day achieved								
PHYSICAL ACTIVITY 30-60 min/day 2pts for every 15 min/day								
PERSONAL GOAL _____ 2pts for each day you meet your goal								
HEALTHY FATS 1 pt/item/day, 4pts max • eat healthy fats including 1 serving of nuts daily • avoid all trans fats • limit saturated fat (less than 7% of cal.) • eat a food high in n-3 fatty acids (flax meal 1T, walnuts 1oz., fish 2oz., canola oil 1T)								
HEALTHY CARBOHYDRATES 1 pt/item/day, 4pts max • eat 5+ servings of fruits and vegetables • eat 3+ servings of whole grains (1 slice bread, 1/2 C dry cereal) • eat a serving (1/2C) of legumes or tofu • limit high glycemic foods (pop, white bread, French fries, white rice, pastry, etc.)								
HEALTHY WEIGHT 4 pts for each day you follow a healthy, low calorie eating plan								

TOTAL WELLNESS POINTS THIS WEEK: _____

TOTAL MILES WALKED THIS WEEK: _____

Personal Wellness Log — Week 6

	SUN	MON	TUE	WED	THU	FRI	SAT	T
SLEEP 7-8 hrs/day 2pts for each day achieved								
WATER 6-8 glasses/day 2pts for every day achieved								
PHYSICAL ACTIVITY 30-60 min/day 2pts for every 15 min/day								
PERSONAL GOAL _____ 2pts for each day you meet your goal								
HEALTHY FATS 1 pt/item/day, 4pts max • eat healthy fats including 1 serving of nuts daily • avoid all trans fats • limit saturated fat (less than 7% of cal.) • eat a food high in n-3 fatty acids (flax meal 1T, walnuts 1oz., fish 2oz., canola oil 1T)								
HEALTHY CARBOHYDRATES 1 pt/item/day, 4pts max • eat 5+ servings of fruits and vegetables • eat 3+ servings of whole grains (1 slice bread, 1/2 C dry cereal) • eat a serving (1/2C) of legumes or tofu • limit high glycemic foods (pop, white bread, French fries, white rice, pastry, etc.)								
HEALTHY WEIGHT 4 pts for each day you follow a healthy, low calorie eating plan								

TOTAL WELLNESS POINTS THIS WEEK: _____

TOTAL MILES WALKED THIS WEEK: _____

Personal Wellness Log — Week 7

	SUN	MON	TUE	WED	THU	FRI	SAT	T
SLEEP 7-8 hrs/day 2pts for each day achieved								
WATER 6-8 glasses/day 2pts for every day achieved								
PHYSICAL ACTIVITY 30-60 min/day 2pts for every 15 min/day								
PERSONAL GOAL _____ 2pts for each day you meet your goal								
HEALTHY FATS 1 pt/item/day, 4pts max • eat healthy fats including 1 serving of nuts daily • avoid all trans fats • limit saturated fat (less than 7% of cal.) • eat a food high in n-3 fatty acids (flax meal 1T, walnuts 1oz., fish 2oz., canola oil 1T)								
HEALTHY CARBOHYDRATES 1 pt/item/day, 4pts max • eat 5+ servings of fruits and vegetables • eat 3+ servings of whole grains (1 slice bread, 1/2 C dry cereal) • eat a serving (1/2C) of legumes or tofu • limit high glycemic foods (pop, white bread, French fries, white rice, pastry, etc.)								
HEALTHY WEIGHT 4 pts for each day you follow a healthy, low calorie eating plan								

TOTAL WELLNESS POINTS THIS WEEK: _____

TOTAL MILES WALKED THIS WEEK: _____

Personal Wellness Log — Week 8

	SUN	MON	TUE	WED	THU	FRI	SAT	T
SLEEP 7-8 hrs/day 2pts for each day achieved								
WATER 6-8 glasses/day 2pts for every day achieved								
PHYSICAL ACTIVITY 30-60 min/day 2pts for every 15 min/day								
PERSONAL GOAL _____ 2pts for each day you meet your goal								
HEALTHY FATS 1 pt/item/day, 4pts max • eat healthy fats including 1 serving of nuts daily • avoid all trans fats • limit saturated fat (less than 7% of cal.) • eat a food high in n-3 fatty acids (flax meal 1T, walnuts 1oz., fish 2oz., canola oil 1T)								
HEALTHY CARBOHYDRATES 1 pt/item/day, 4pts max • eat 5+ servings of fruits and vegetables • eat 3+ servings of whole grains (1 slice bread, 1/2 C dry cereal) • eat a serving (1/2C) of legumes or tofu • limit high glycemic foods (pop, white bread, French fries, white rice, pastry, etc.)								
HEALTHY WEIGHT 4 pts for each day you follow a healthy, low calorie eating plan								

TOTAL WELLNESS POINTS THIS WEEK:_____

TOTAL MILES WALKED THIS WEEK: _____

Personal Wellness Log — ONGOING

Health indicator	Starting value	Desirable values	My Goal	Achieved by (date)
Weight	_____		_____	_____
BMI	_____	BMI <25	_____	_____
Waist girth	_____	M <37, F <32	_____	_____
Exercise	_____		_____	_____
min/wk, or	_____	150+ min/wk	_____	_____
miles/wk, or	_____	6-15+ miles/wk	_____	_____
steps/day	_____	6,000-10,000+	_____	_____
Blood pressure	_____	<120/80	_____	_____
Cholesterol	_____	<200	_____	_____
Other	_____		_____	_____

NOTES:

_____

_____

_____

_____

_____

_____

NOTES:

Let's Move Exercises

The recommendation is a minimum of 30 minutes of moderate exercise for six days a week. A rule of thumb to understand moderate exercise is exercise that causes you to break a sweat or exercise during which you cannot sing but can still have a conversation. For a more technical grasp of moderate exercise, one can aim at achieving at least 75 percent of their maximum heart rate. To find this out, just subtract your age from 220; the number remaining is the maximum heart rate. Now the goal is to achieve 75 percent of that number. Let's say that you are twenty years old. Your maximum heart rate would be 200, but the desired heart rate to achieve would be 75 percent of 200, which would be 150. An adequate exercise program should include exercises aimed at improving cardiorespiratory fitness, as well as muscular strength, flexibility, and balance.

OBTAINING 30 MINUTES of Moderate Physical Exercise daily could add years to your life.

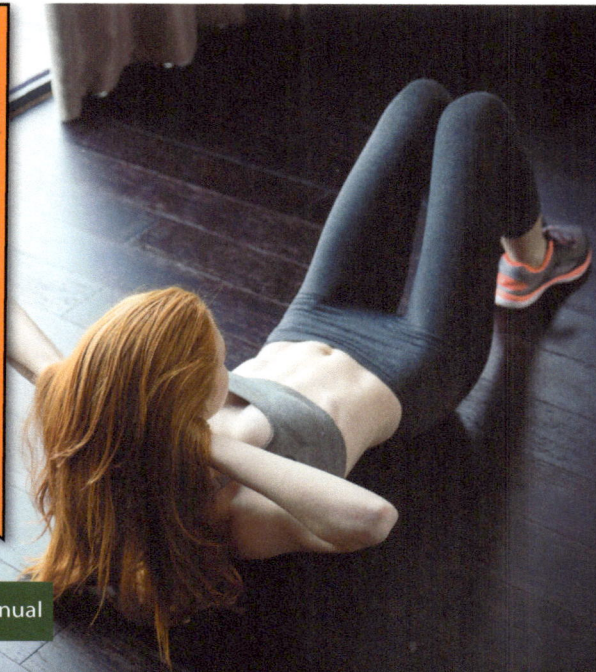

Push Up to Plank

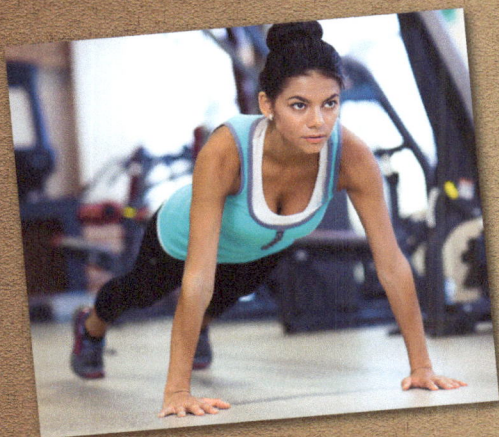

**Classification:
Strength & Stabilization**

Technique: Begin laying face down with hands at chest level, slightly wider than shoulder width apart. Extend arm and perform press with arms fully extended, hips neutral, and back straight. Keep pectorals and shoulders engaged at top of push up. Lower back to bottom position and repeat for 10-20 reps. Avoid dropping the head, rounding of mid-spine, or elevating shoulders to ears.

Optional: at the last rep lower down into plank position with elbows on the ground with hands parallel, straight head, and toes on the ground. Hold for 10-30 Seconds or as long as possible. Avoid dropping the head, rounding of mid-spine, or elevating shoulders to ears.

Cool down: Ten minute walk, bike, or row.

Medicine Ball Lift and Chop

Technique: Stand with feet hip width apart. Hold medicine ball in both hands at left hip. Drop into quarter squat. Begin standing up extending the knees and hips. At the same time extend medicine ball over head in a diagonal motion. The end of the motion should have the medicine ball over the right shoulder. Complete 10-20 reps and switch sides.

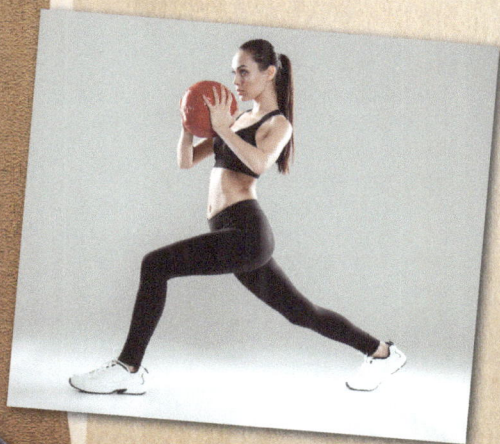

**Classification:
Strength**

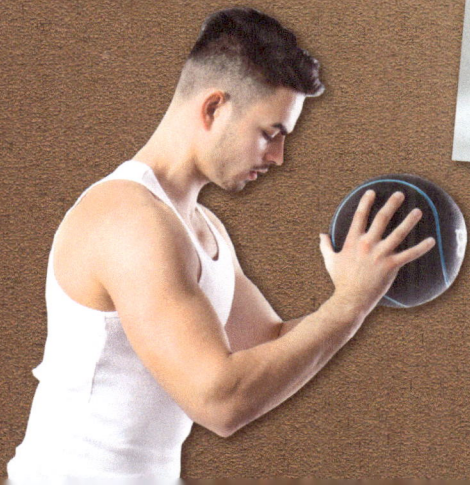

Ice Skaters

Technique: Stand on one leg. Hop from side to side alternating legs as if you were jumping over a tree branch. Pump your arms side to side reaching above shoulder no higher than head (opposite hand to the standing leg), Knees are slightly bent and body is low. Repeat for 10-20 Reps

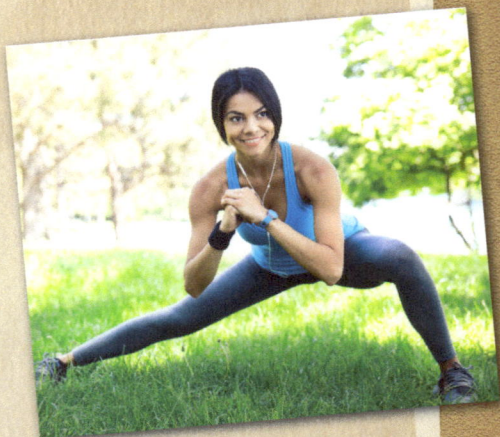

**Classification:
Reactive Power**

Body Weight Squat

Warm up: Cardiovascular: Complete a 20 Minute walk, bike, or row at a low - moderate pace.

Technique: Stand in a shoulder width stance with toes pointed straight ahead. Keeping an upright trunk/torso. Bending hips back and bending knees will initiate the squat. Lower as far as body can be controlled form, goal is to be at or lower than knee level. Extend the hips, knees, and ankles to return to standing position.

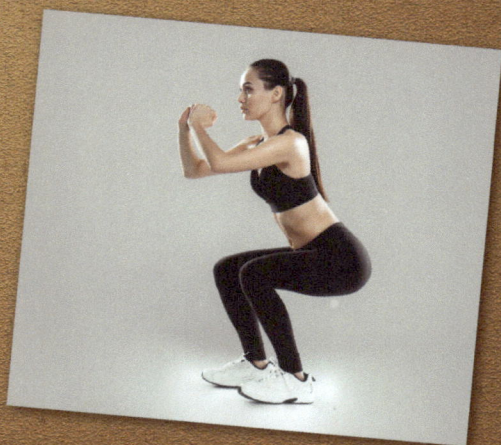

**Classification:
Strength**

Triceps Dip

Sit on chair, knees bent, hands grasping seat. Walk feet forward until butt is off seat. Bend elbows, lowering hips. Press back up, straightening arms.

Make it easier: Skip dips. Sit on chair, holding one dumbbell in both hands overhead. Bend elbows, lowering weight behind head. Straighten arms, pressing weight overhead.

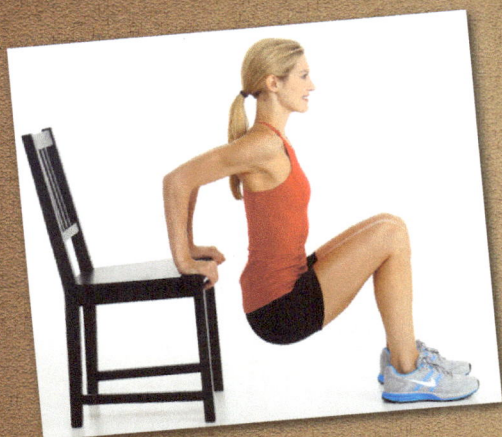

**Targets:
triceps & shoulders**

Alternating Forward Lunge with Hammer Curl

Stand holding dumbbells by sides. Step forward with right leg and slowly lower into a lunge while curling weights toward shoulders. Press into right foot and return to start, lowering weights. Alternate front leg with each rep.

Make it easier:
Do lunges without weights.

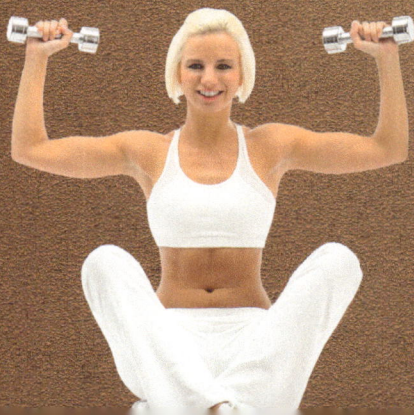

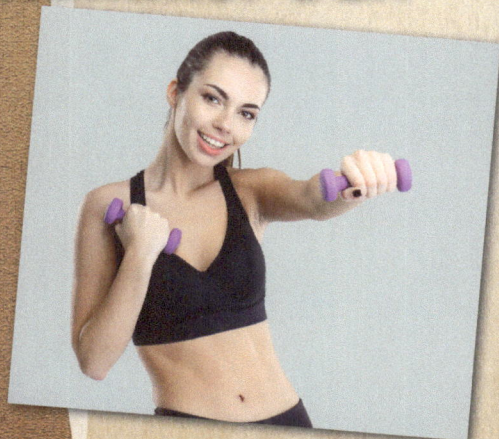

**Targets:
butt, legs & biceps**

Knee Push-Up

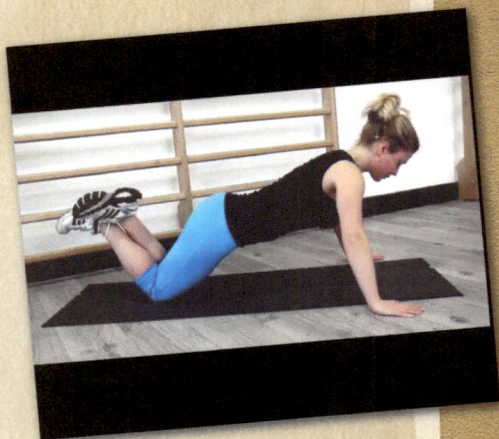

Start in modified push-up position, knees on floor. Keeping abs tight, bend elbows and lower chest toward floor. Press back up to start and extend right arm at shoulder level. Continue alternating arms with each rep.

Make it easier: Omit the punch.

**Targets:
chest, shoulders,
arms & core**

POWER MOVE: Split Jump

Start in a shallow lunge, right foot 2 to 3 feet in front of left foot. Jump up and, while in the air, scissor-kick so you land with left leg forward, immediately lowering into a shallow lunge. Alternate front leg with each rep.

Make it easier: Skip jumps, do alternating lunges.

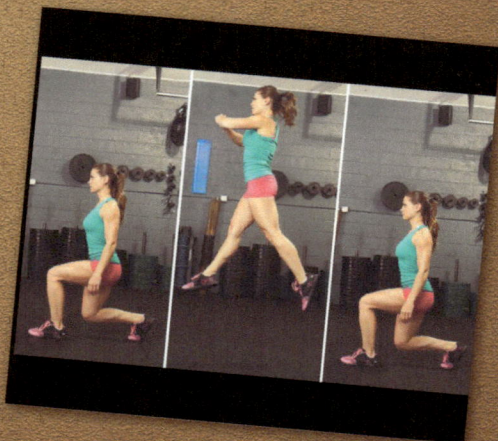

Targets: butt & legs
(and boosts heart rate!)

Wall Leg Squat

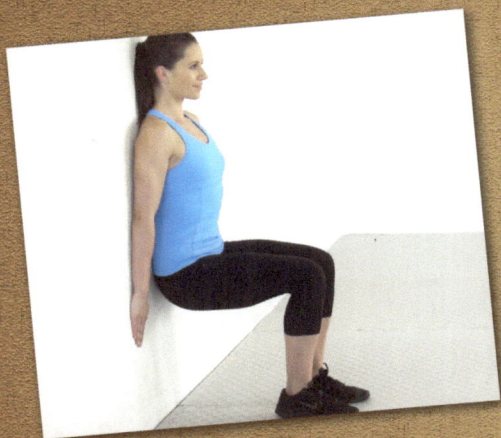

Stand straight with your legs slightly wider than your shoulders and point your toes outward.

Once positioned, focus your balance on your heals and squat down as seen in image. Drop till your knees are at a 90 degree angle.

Execute 10-20 reps per set. As muscular strength/endurance increases the sets and reps can be modified.

Push Up

Get in a push up position, but support your body weight on your elbows directly beneath your shoulders. Keep your feet flexed with bottoms of toes on the floor.

Clasp hands in front of your face, so your forearms make a "v" shape.

Rise up on your toes and forearms leaving your body hovering above the floor a few inches.

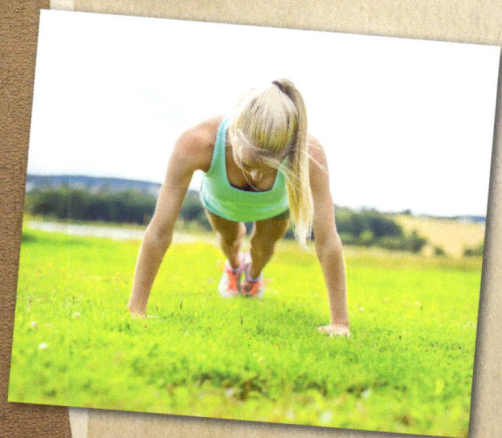

Draw your navel toward your spine and tighten your butt. Keep your head relaxed by looking at the floor.

Hold position for 10-15 seconds and lower yourself back to the floor.

Plank

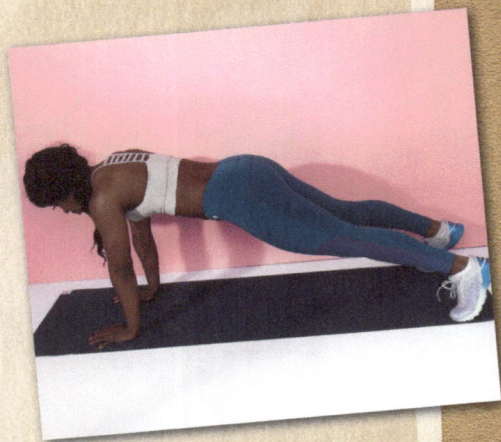

Get into a high plank position. Keep your back flat and firmly place hands on the ground, shoulder width apart.

Begin to lower body—keeping your back flat and eyes focus on a focal point—until arms are at a 90 degree angle. If needed, lower body till chest touches the floor.

Push up and contract chest muscle at the top. Repeat 10-12 reps per set. Modify amount according to your physical fitness.

Butt Lift (Bridge)

Lie flat on the floor on your back with your hands by your sides and knees bent. Your feet should be shoulder width apart. This is the starting position

Push primarily with your heels, lift your hips off the floor while keeping your back straight. Once at the top, hold position for a second.

Slowly go back down to the starting position.

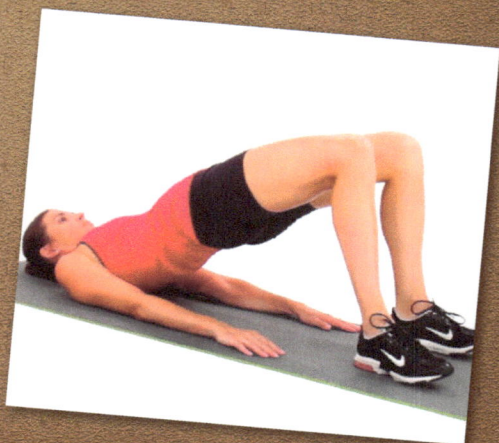

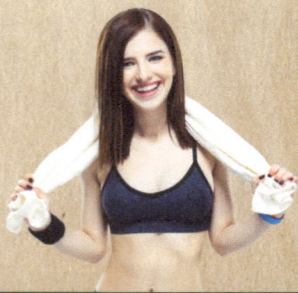

Walking Lunges

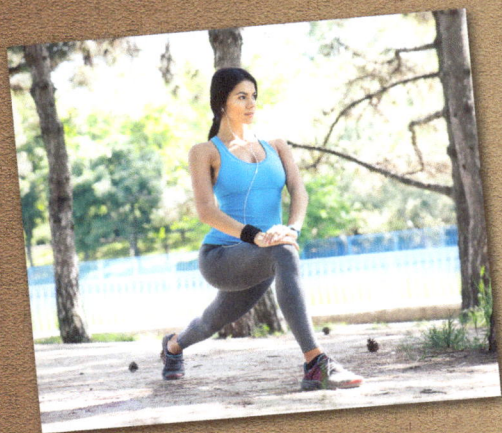

Begin movement standing with legs at hip distance. Take a large step forward with your right knee, as you move downward with your right knee at 90 degrees (do not let knee pass over front of right foot), your left knee should come near touching the ground. Push and return to standing position and repeat with your left leg leading.

Chest Pass Rotation

Begin by standing with your body turned at a 90 degree angle from a wall. Place feet shoulder width apart and pointed straight. Hold medicine ball with both hands at chest level with your elbows flexed. Initiate the movement by contracting your glutes and rotate your body quickly toward the wall, pivoting your back leg as your body turns. Use your entire upper body to push and release the ball toward to the wall as hard as possible. Do not allow your shoulders to shrug as your throw the ball. Catch the ball and repeat as quickly as possible with form.

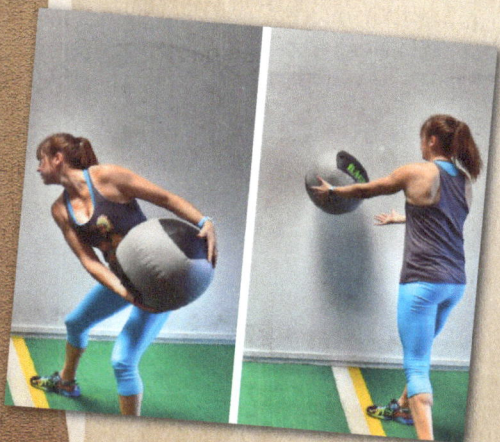

Multiplanar Step Up

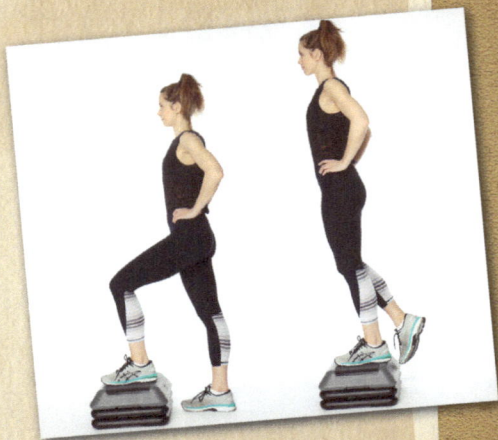

Begin by standing in front of a box or platform with feet shoulders-width apart and pointing straight ahead (hips should be in a neutral position). Lift one leg directly beside balance leg, hop up and land on top of box on one leg. Hold for 3-5 seconds. Repeat.

Advanced: Use the same format to hop forward and lateral (left and right).

Single Leg Romanian Deadlift

Begin by standing with feet shoulders-width apart and pointing straight ahead (hips should be in a neutral position). Lift one leg directly beside balance leg, bend from the waist and slowly reach hand down toward the toes of the balance leg (Keep the spine in a neutral position and avoid hunching over). Slowly stand upright activating abdominal muscles and gluteal muscles. Repeat with opposite leg.

Advanced: Add light dumbbells.

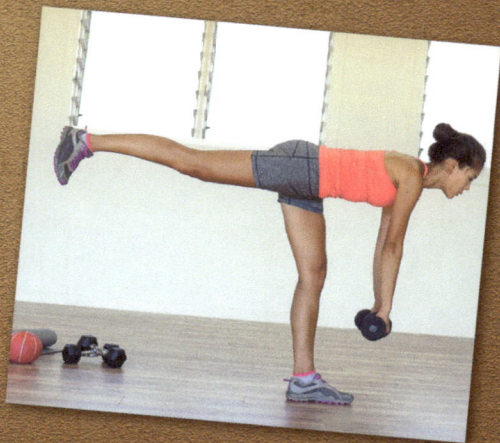

Squat to Press

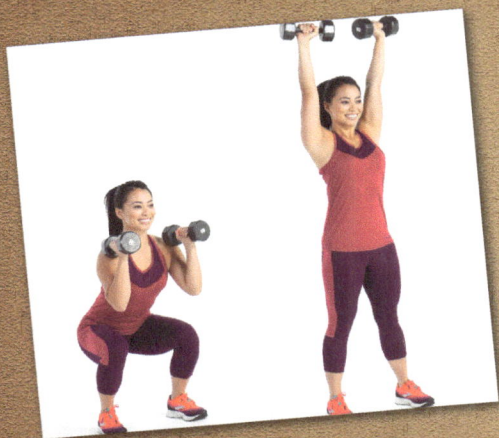

Start by standing with your feet shoulder-width apart with dumbbells above your shoulders. Squat down keeping your back flat and your knees over your toes. (Goal for Gluteus to end up at parallel with knees or below). Push through your heels to return to standing while pressing the dumbbells overhead with arms fully extended. Return to starting position and repeat.

**Targets:
Gluteus, Hamstring,
Quadriceps & Shoulders**

Plank with Alternating Shoulder Taps

Start by getting into a pushup position with your hands shoulder-width apart on the floor and your legs straight back and arms fully extended. Keeping your hips square to the floor, lift your right hand and tap your left shoulder. Make sure Gluteus and Core do not drop towards ground and body remains in a straight position. Return to start and repeat with the other arm. Sets can be done for time or repetitions.

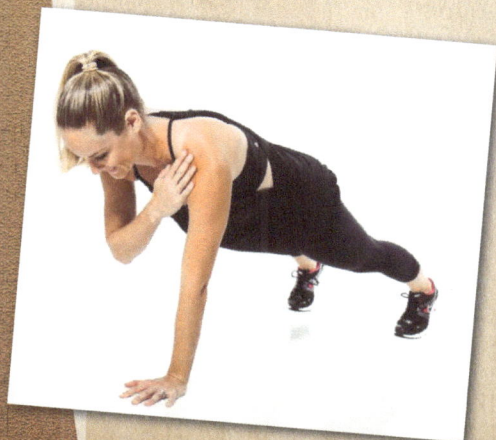

Targets: Core, Shoulders, Gluteus, Hamstring, Quadriceps & Shoulders

Scissor Kick

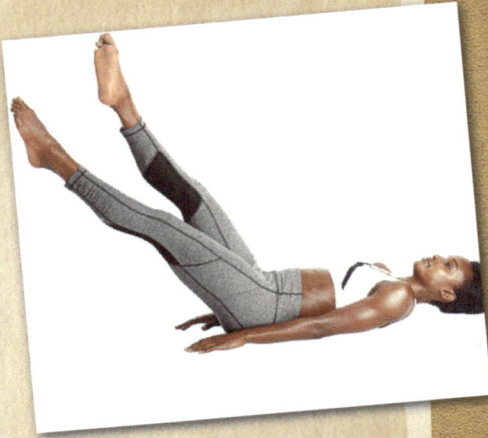

Start by Laying on your back with your legs extended in front of you and your arms by your side, palms down. Keeping your legs straight with your knees slightly bent, lift one leg upward until it is at a 45 degree angle and your toe is pointing to the ceiling. Lower the leg that is raised while raising the other leg that is lowered, keeping your heels a few inches off the ground at all times. Breathing regularly, continue to alternate legs in this scissor motion. Sets can be done for time or repetitions.

**Targets:
Core**

Bent Over Dumbbell Row

Start with a dumbbell in each hand palms facing body, bend knees slightly and bring your torso forward by bending at the waist; make sure to keep your back straight until it is almost parallel to the floor. The weights should hang directly in front of you as your arms hang perpendicular to the floor and your torso. While keeping the torso stationary, lift the dumbbells to your side (exhale), keeping the elbows close to the body. On the top of movement, squeeze the back muscles. Slowly lower the weight again to the starting position as you inhale. Repeat for the recommended amount of repetitions.

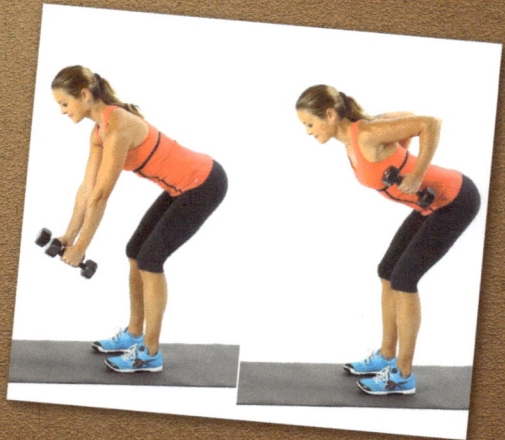

Targets: Middle Trapezius and Rhomboids, Biceps & Erector Spinae

NOTES:

Fitness Planning Worksheet

Activities I want to include in my fitness program:

- ❏ Walking
- ❏ Jogging
- ❏ Cycling/Biking
- ❏ Swimming
- ❏ Running

- ❏ Squatting
- ❏ Crunches
- ❏ Weight Lifting
- ❏ Hiking
- ❏ Other _____

Duration (time per session): _____

Time of day I plan on exercising: _____

Frequency (times per week): _____

Intensity: ❏ Easy pace ❏ Moderate pace ❏ Vigorous pace

Aerobic miles per week:

- ❏ 6 aerobic miles per week
- ❏ 10 aerobic miles per week
- ❏ 15 aerobic miles per week
- ❏ 20 aerobic miles per week

Total aerobic miles per week: _____
Number of steps daily: _____
(if using pedometer)

My Goal (goal to achieve in 6 to 10 weeks)
Write out and be specific: _____
_____
_____
_____

Reward for reaching my goal: _____
_____

Physical Activity Log

Wk	Mon	Tue	Wed	Thu	Fri	Sat	Sun	Week's total aerobic miles	Weight
1									
2									
3									
4									
5									
6									
7									
8									

NOTES:

_____

_____

_____

_____

_____

_____

_____

_____

_____

_____

_____

_____

_____

_____

_____

_____

_____

_____

_____

_____

_____

CONCLUSION

Without a doubt, there are many challenges that we face every day, in the family, work and personal spaces. It is for this reason that through this Manual of Exercises and Nutrition I have tried to contribute in some way, to facilitate your lifestyle, sharing healthy recipes and practical exercises that put into practice will help improve your health.

Remember that health is "A choice, not a destiny," therefore; persevere every day until you strengthen your good eating habits and the regular practice of physical exercise. If you and your family incorporate these good practices, you can experience their benefits not only in the present, but in the future you can enjoy a better quality of life.

www.ingramcontent.com/pod-product-compliance
Lightning Source LLC
Chambersburg PA
CBHW041215270326
41930CB00001B/25